Keto Meal Plans
and
Much More

Shopping Lists, 30-Day Plan, Vegetarian, Vegan, Mediterranean, Affordable Guide with Amazing Results, for 50 Years Above

Disclaimer

The information in this book is for educational purposes only. It should not be taken as a direct advice from medical care personnel. The advice from your physician remains the best source of information. Therefore, always seek medical advice from your doctor to ascertain if your body or health condition allows for keto diet meal plan like the ones in this eBook.

All the meal plans in this book are approved by dieticians. They are healthy and can give you the best results a keto diet can offer. But they may not be suitable for all individuals without some modifications on your part.

I made sure that you get the best meal plan you can find, but consultation with your doctor is required before you start. It is your responsibility to evaluate and confirm the information in my ebook with other good sources. Remember to get the involvement of your physician or any qualified medical health care professional before you embark on the keto diet journey.

TABLE OF CONTENTS

CHAPTER ONE

Introduction

When you search health and fitness online sites, what do you see? You see various articles and products suggesting amazing diets and ways to reduce weight. Among all this helpful information, keto diet towers high and is becoming popular in recent times. Many grownups or adults are turning to keto for solutions to body fat or for easing some health problems.

Keto diet is a form of food plan that reduces carbs intake while increasing fats and protein to help the body burn unwanted fat. Apart from fat burning, keto diet helps the body to lose weight and enhances overall health. Even people with type 2 diabetes can use keto to curb the symptoms of their condition.

Keto diet is good for men and women who are 50 years and above as long as they do not have health issues. One of the great benefits keto offers to this age group is weight loss. One thing to always keep in mind is that you need to choose the healthiest among in the food list. Create a balance of veggies, unprocessed carbs, and lean meat when making your keto selection. Stick to whole foods due to their ability to sustain the body for a longer period.

CHAPTER TWO

Week 1 Meal Plan and Shopping List

The main goal of this book is to help you stick to the simplest possible plan. Simplicity is key when it comes to keto meal plan, for there is no point struggling throughout the duration. Since you are about to go on low-carb diet for a while, it is necessary to make a smooth transition. This aspect is necessary because you may have a hard time overcoming your usual carbs cravings.

You may get the early signs of ketosis which is called "morning flu" and these include fatigue, headache, and brain fogginess. Try as much as you can to drink lots of water and do not forget adding a little salt. You will pee all the time due to the diuretic ability of the keto diet. When you pee, you are flushing out electrolytes, which will trigger a thumping headache. Keep your salt and water intake high, and you will have nothing to worry.

When you drink water, try to add a sprinkle of salt in it. At least 4 liters per day is the recommended quantity. Do not worry about getting high blood pressure due to the intake of water and salt. Recent studies have it that there is no link between sodium and high blood pressure. So relax and plan your keto meal for week one.

Shopping List for Week 1
Veggies
Sugar snap peas
Parsley

Green beans

Oranges

Lots of Spinach

1 green pepper

6 lemons

3 onions

Broccoli

Cauliflower

Sauces

Red wine

Chicken stock

Soy sauce

Coconut milk

Tomato sauce

Beef broth

Rao's tomato sauce

Gluten-free red boat fish sauce

Dijon mustard

Worcestershire

Full fat ranch dressing

Meat

Shrimp

Eggs

Stew meat

Bacon

Chorizo sausage

Chicken thighs

Ground beef

Canned chicken

Pork rinds

Bacon and cheddar

Fats

Pecans

Coconut oil

Bottled olive oil

Bacon fat (saved from your cooked bacon)

Heavy cream

Unsalted butter

Cheese

Parmesan

Cheese

Cheddar cheese

Queso fresco cheese

Spices

Thyme

Bay leaf

Black pepper

Cardamom

Paprika

Sage

Chives

Oregano

Cumin

Salt

Ginger

Chili pepper

Rosemary

Yellow curry powder

Xanthan gum

Cayenne pepper

Week 1 Meal Plan

Breakfast

For your breakfast, get something tasty, easy, and can have leftovers. It will be great if you start your first week on a weekend. With that, you will have enough time to prepare a meal that will last an entire week. You may even call a relation or friend to come over and help you make a great keto meal for your first week. Remember, the rule is simplicity and nothing more, so you don't have to make it hard for yourself by preparing it during weekdays.

Lunch

Keep it simple during lunch, and you may prepare something like salad and meat carefully dressed in high fat. To avoid making it too expensive, you may use the leftover of the previous night. If you have canned chicken or fish, that would be a great option. If you have access to canned meat only, read the label carefully to make sure there are little or no additives.

Dinner

Your dinner time should be a combination of some meat and leafy greens such as spinach and broccoli. The meal should contain high fat, with moderate addition of protein. Keep in mind that to avoid dessert for the first two weeks at least.

CHAPTER THREE

Week 2 Meal Plan and Shopping List

Once week one is over, your resolve to continue should be stronger. By now your experience should move from difficult to easy. For the second week, you are not going to keep it simple especially for breakfast. This time, you will introduce what you may call the ketoproof coffee. It is a mixture of butter, heavy cream, and coconut oil in coffee. Wait. Before you say you don't like it, try it first. The concoction may sound strange but it is a combination of the butter you already know blended in oil and cream to give your coffee some kind of richness that you will absolutely love.

Shopping List for Week 2

Vegetables

Lemons

Spring onion

Green beans

Mushrooms

Sugar snap peas

Cheese

Blue cheddar cheese

Cheddar cheese

Mozzarella

Cream cheese

Meat

Chorizo sausage

Chicken breast

Spices

Baking soda

Baking powder

Tone's southwest chipotle seasoning

Mrs. Dash table blend

Sauces

Coffee

Yellow mustard

Hit sauce

Apple cider vinegar

Crunch

Pecans

Almonds

Pork rinds

Special Items

Milled flax seed

Almond flour

Week 2 Meal Plan

Breakfast

You will bring in that keto proof coffee or if you don't like it with coffee, use tea. It is rare not to like the taste of the amazing drink. But if you think you don't still like the sound and sight of it, try eating the ingredients separately but at the same time.

Perhaps a good explanation of the advantages of keto proof coffee will help you see things differently. It is always good to be sure of every meal you have planned to take before going into keto dieting. This way, you are fully prepared to follow through any meal plan you set for yourself.

Advantages of Ketoproof Coffee
- Ketoproof diet contains medium-chain triglycerides that lead to a reduction of the adipose tissue or fat tissue in the body.
- It contains fat that leads to an increased amount of energy, effective weight loss, and more efficiency in

daily activities. Fat is the main component of keto proof coffee.

- Medium-chain fatty acids or MCFAs help to increase the energy the body expends. These MCFAs convert to ketones and the body absorbs them better than regular oils.

Think of adding a little sweetener if you are not comfortable with the taste. Choose vanilla, cinnamon, or stevia extract or whatever you feel will give it a great taste. To spice up to the drink, you may take these sweeteners in turns each day.

If this will be your first time taking keto proof coffee, try drinking it slowly, taking between 1-2 hours to sip until you gulp it down. Too much exposure to coconut can make you run to the toilet often, so it is safe to take your time while drinking ketoproof coffee.

Lunch

Simplicity still continues for your lunch, and you are going with the previous meat you had on the last day of the first week. Combine it with green veggies, tastily dressed with fat or vinaigrettes. Keep the right amount of fat and protein throughout your meals and don't go beyond the recommended quantity.

Dinner

Your dinner should be made up of meat, high-fat dressings, and veggies. Since you are still early in your keto journey, add a slathering of butter to give it a great taste. Do not eat dessert yet, as this is week two.

CHAPTER FOUR

Week 3 Meal Plan and Shopping List

You are going to make a slight change in your meal plan. In the morning, eat as much fat as the diet allows and fast throughout the day until dinner time. This method has a lot of health benefits you may not be aware of right now. Also, you get to rest more without having to cook and prepare meals all the time. It will be helpful if you drink your breakfast in the morning (7am) and eat dinner in the evening (7pm).

During fasting, your body has enough time to break down fats stored for energy. In ketosis, the body imitates a fasting state by using the fats in the body due to the absence of glucose in the bloodstream. While on an intermittent fast, the body uses stored fat instead of the fat you are eating at the moment. It may sound great but you should know that you need to keep eating fat to avoid going into a mode of starvation.

Intermittent fasting has a lot of benefits which include longevity, mental clarity, and blood lipids levels. If you cannot go with the fasting, follow week one meal plan.

Shopping List for Week 3
Vegetables
Lemons

Sauces
Spicy brown mustard
Red wine vinegar
Liquid smoke

Sugar-free maple syrup

Pesto sauce

Gluten-free fish sauce or red boat fish
sauce

Meat

Chicken thighs

Boneless, skinless

Pork tenderloin

Spices

Nutmeg

Dried sage

Instant coffee ground

Ground clove

Vanilla

Dried rosemary

Cheese

Mozzarella cheese or halloumi cheese

Special Item

Liquid stevia

Erythritol

Breakfast

Week three is full-fat foods during breakfast just like in week 2, but you are going to double the quantity of ketoproof coffee or tea you drink. You should add all the ingredients twice as much as before. That means more coconut, more butter, and more heavy cream. That is a lot of calories already, isn't it? It will keep you full until dinner time. You should not forget to drink enough water to keep your body hydrated.

Lunch

You don't need lunch. Yes, NO LUNCH for you this time because the morning meal should keep you energized and full until evening. You may feel hungry at around

2pm but with enough water to drink, you can stay that way until dinner time.

Dinner

During your long-awaited dinner, you should serve meat, veggies, and fats on your table. But guess what is coming in now? Dessert! Yes, remember you start eating dessert in week 3 to make your meal look and taste great. So this week is all about having a tasty meal, in addition to a good treat, and weight loss. Wow, lucky you!

CHAPTER FIVE

Week 4 Meal Plan and Shopping List

Things are getting stricter this time, and fasting is still going on. After a full week of intermittent fast, it is time to skip breakfast and lunch. Yes, you heard it right: breakfast and lunch are going out for a while. Keep drinking water and take a little salt with it. You may take tea, coffee, or flavored water of your choice as long as they don't break the rules of the diet. Avoid thinking about your stomach or you may hear it growling loudly in your ears.

If you feel that this type of fasting is difficult for you, go back and follow week 2 meal plan. There is nothing wrong with that decision if that is your choice.

However, if you can fast, soon you will discover that your body will adjust to it and you will reap the health benefits of intermittent fasting.

Shopping List for Week 4

Crunch

Pistachios

Peanuts or the butter

Pumpkin seeds

Spices

Red food coloring

Five-spice

Capers

Fats

Sesame oil

Meat

Ground chicken

Sauces

Rice vinegar

Chili garlic paste

Reduced sugar ketchup

1 can Coors light

Cheese

Mozzarella cheese

Cream cheese

Blue cheese crumbles

Meal Plan for Week 4
Breakfast

Fasting continues and you may drink coffee if you like caffeine. Tea is another option if coffee is not your thing. Like coffee, tea can give your body a whole lot of benefits.

Lunch

Drink water, drink more and keep drinking water from breakfast time to dinner time. Since you don't get to eat lunch, you need to keep yourself hydrated. Remember the quantity of water per day should be 4 liters.

Dinner

Now the time you are waiting for has come. Dinner time! You can't wait to have your dessert with lots of food. You may take the recommended snack first before going for your actual meal.

Takeaway

Follow the meal plan for each week and you can start all over again from week one to week four for your week 5 and so on. For those who do not like pork rinds, you can use blue cheese dressing, ground chicken thighs, or lamb as long as it is low-carb. You can use turkey bacon in the place of regular bacon, and higher varieties of beef are another good option. You may substitute spinach for lettuce if that is fine with you.

Within four weeks of going on this diet, some people lose up to 20 or 40 pounds. Sometimes, you may have mood swings or feel emotional in the process. But that is nothing to worry about as your body will adjust to it soon and your mood will get better.

If the whole family is doing the keto diet together, you need to multiply the amount of food by the number of people in the family. For instance, if you live with your daughter, partner, or grandson, or you are a family of four, just multiply the quantity of food by the number of persons. The meal plan is meant to guide you on what to do and what to expect each week.

If you are not comfortable with coconut oil, use avocado oil, ghee, olive oil, or macadamia as good substitutes. Creamy dressing or vinaigrette is also good replacements for salad dressings. If caffeine is a problem, you can avoid drinking coffee and choose caffeine-free tea or decaf coffee. Some people go for bulletproof cocoa but it is a matter of choice. If you are allergic to nuts, consider using almond seed flour, pumpkin seed flour or sunflower seed flour.

CHAPTER SIX

Keto Diet for Vegetarians

If you are a vegetarian, you can go on a keto diet that fits into your eating habits. A vegetarian diet is considered by many as one of the world's healthiest diet. Eating vegetarian foods will have a lot of benefits such as reduced risks of diabetes and heart disease. These amazing benefits are why many vegetarians love their lifestyle even though a vegetarian keto diet or even vegetarian diet may not the best diet in the world.

Research has shown that a keto diet is more effective than an ordinary vegetarian diet when it comes to weight loss, blood sugar, and enhancing triglycerides levels. It can also reduce the effects of type 2 diabetes, polycystic ovary syndrome, epilepsy, obesity, and certain cancer. But the environmental danger of keto is a source of growing concern. Dairy and meat come from animals reared in controlled environments. They are low in nutrition, and contribute to climate change in addition to posing a direct abuse of animals.

However, we can solve this problem by taking some principles from both keto diet and vegetarian diet. We can create the perfect diet plan by choosing our sources carefully. This is how to create a meal plan that combines a ketogenic diet and a vegetarian diet in one diet without upsetting the balance in nature. The name of the diet is simply a vegetarian ketogenic diet.

Vegetarian Keto Diet Explained

A vegetarian keto diet is a diet that does not contain fowl flesh, meat, and fish. This form of diet gives you all the benefits of keto diet while at the same time cutting down on carbs intake. Dairy and eggs are two main nutrient-dense products from animals you can add to your vegetarian keto diet. But if you don't like the idea and do not want to affect the environment in any way, you can source these two products from cows and chicken raised in pastures.

Here are rules for vegetarian keto dieting:

1. Eat enough low-carb vegetables.
2. Eliminate meat, poultry, and fish from your daily meal.
3. About 70% of your overall calories should be made up of fats.

4. Find a reliable keto calculator to measure the right amount of macros and calories you need.

5. Eat proteins from plants, high-fat dairy, and egg.

6. Set your carbs limit to 35 grams.

7. When necessary, use supplements such as zinc, iron, DHA & EPA, and D3.

A Sample Meal Plan for Vegetarians

Monday

For breakfast, take 1 or 2 slices of bread (Zucchini bread and walnuts are recommended), and add cream cheese or butter.

Lunch should be made up of 1 great serving fried goat cheese salad and charred vegetables.

For dinner, 5 minutes keto pizza will do for
the evening

Extra Dish: Asparagus fries and some red
pepper aioli.

Tuesday

Breakfast: a serving of fluffy buttermilk

Lunch: keto mug lasagna

Dinner: eggplant and bacon alfredo

Extra Dish: a serving of keto creamed
spinach

Wednesday

Breakfast: pumpkin spiced French toast

Lunch: One or two servings of spinach with
herb and feta wraps

Dinner: one or two servings of roasted red bell pepper and cauliflower

Extra Dish: one serving of keto tater tots

Thursday

Breakfast: One or two servings of cinnamon roll oatmeal

Lunch: Two or three servings of garlic and herb monkey bread

Dinner: One or two servings of avocado-walnut and Zucchini ribbons

Extra Dish: One serving of cheesy cauliflower casserole

Friday

Breakfast: one serving of pumpkin-spiced French toast

Lunch: One serving of fried goat cheese salad and charred vegetables

Dinner: One serving of bacon alfredo and eggplant

Extra Dish: One serving of red pepper aioli and asparagus fries

Saturday

Breakfast: One or two slices of keto Zucchini bread, walnut, with cream cheese or butter

Lunch: One or two servings of cauliflower soup with roasted red bell pepper

Dinner: One serving of five minutes keto pizza

Extra Dish: One serving of cheesy cauliflower casserole

Sunday

Breakfast: one serving of fluffy buttermilk pancakes

Lunch: one serving of keto mug lasagna

Dinner: one or two servings of avocado-walnut and Zucchini ribbons

How to Reduce Your Carb Intake on Vegetarian Keto Diet

Most vegetarians often eat too many carbs when on a keto diet. This is a common mistake that should be controlled for better results. The reason is that carbohydrates foods are among the favorites for many vegetarians. Some of the most loved high-carbs foods are:

Fruits: bananas, oranges, apples, and many others

Grains: wheat, corn, cereal, rice, and others

Tubers: yams, potatoes, etc

Legumes: peas, black beans, lentils, etc

Sugar: syrup, maple agave, honey, etc

Avoid the food listed above when you are on a keto diet. They are high-carb foods and even one serving of any of them can exceed the keto carb limit and ruin your ketosis. But that does not mean you have no good alternatives to fall back on. There are other foods to take apart from eggs and lettuce.

Here is a list of good options for a healthy vegetarian keto diet you can eat:

Leafy greens: kale, spinach

Nuts and seeds: pumpkin seeds, almonds, pistachio, sunflower seeds

Vegan meats: seitan, tofu, tempeh, high-protein, low-carb meat (vegan)

Sweeteners: monk fruit, stevia, erythritol, other low-carb sweeteners

Other fats: olive oil, MCT oil, coconut oil, avocado oil, etc

Vegetables (above ground): cauliflower, broccoli, zucchini

High-fat eggs and dairy: high-fat cream, eggs, butter, hard cheeses, etc

Avocados and berries: blackberries, raspberries, etc

The above diet gives you a balance between being a vegetarian and a keto dieter at the same time. It takes into consideration most of the nutritional needs covering the entire duration of the diet.

CHAPTER SEVEN

Keto Diet for Vegans

The three main points of a vegan diet are climate change, animal suffering, and health. People who follow the vegan diet primarily try to bring solutions to these areas. But some people are skeptical about this diet and wonder if it is possible to practice a vegan lifestyle successfully. The answer to this all-important question is yes. You can be a vegan and it is possible to follow the diet successfully for as long as you want.

Different people have different experiences when they go on a particular diet. While some feel better on a low-carb diet and consume animal products, others feel much better when they eat high-carb vegan foods.

A vegan diet is not the best for people with certain health conditions. For instance, if you are suffering from diabetes type 1, diabetes type 2, epilepsy, obesity, and Parkinson's disease, a vegan diet is not very effective. Following a keto diet is the best way to help or reverse your health condition.

Looking at this, does it mean that vegans should quit their lifestyle and begin to consume animal products? No, not at all. If you are having a hard time following a complete high-carb vegan diet, and you feel that a keto diet will give you what you need, there is a way to combine the best parts of both diets.

Vegan Keto Diet Explained

The vegan keto diet is a highly restrictive food plan. However, it is possible to follow it without encountering problems that will make you quit too soon. If you have been thinking of how to make this work without jeopardizing animals' lives or ruining the environment, here are rules to help you observe it perfectly.

Your total carbs consumption should be 35 grams or less

Get rid of eggs, dairy, fish, meats, and other animal products

Eat a lot of low-carb veggies

Calculate the number of carbs, protein, and fat you consume per day using a keto calculator

Not less than 70% of your total fat calories should come from plants

About 25% of protein calories should be plant-based

When not getting enough nutrients, use supplements such as DHA & EPA, vitamin B6, B12, D3, zinc iron and taurine

What Not to Eat on Vegan Keto Diet
It is already hard enough to reduce carbs intake on a keto diet, now how do you limit your carb intake on a vegan keto diet? Let's look at a simple list of foods you need to avoid on a vegan keto diet.

Fruits: oranges, bananas, apples

Legumes: peas, black beans, lentils

Grains: corn, rice, wheat, cereal

Tubers: yams, potatoes, etc

Sugar: maple syrup, agave, honey

What to Eat on Vegan Keto Diet

Nuts and Seeds: almonds, pumpkin seeds, pistachios, sunflower seeds

Mushrooms: lion's mane, king's oyster, shiitake

Vegan Meats: tofu, seitan, tempeh, high protein/low-carb vegan meats

Alternative High-Fat Dairy: vegan cheeses, coconut cream, unsweetened coconut-based yogurt

Vegetables (above ground): cauliflower, zucchini, broccoli

Avocados and Berries: blackberries, raspberries, low glycemic impact berries

Sea Vegetables: kelp, bladderwrack, dulse,

Leafy Greens: kale, spinach

Sweeteners: monk fruit, stevia, erythritol, low-carb sweeteners

Fermented Foods: kimchi, sauerkraut, Natto

Other Fats: olive oil, avocado oil, coconut oil, MCT oil

What a Vegan Keto Meal Plan Looks Like

Breakfast: peanut butter pancakes with McKeto strawberry milkshake. Add vegan protein powder or prepare a keto-friendly smoothie blended with MCT oil and flavored vegan protein.

Lunch: oven-roasted Caprese salad or crispy tofu and bok choy salad

Dinner: vegetarian red coconut curry with spicy grilled eggplant and mint and parsley or vegan tofu and eggplant or warm Asian broccoli salad as a side or extra dish

Keeping Up with the Vegan Keto Diet
The vegan diet has more plant foods than any other diet but it is not the healthiest diet you can find. Plants do not have most of the nutrients that the body needs to remain healthy. According to studies, vegans are prone to deficiencies in vitamins K2, D, A, and in B12, calcium, zinc, iron, and EPA & DHA. To reduce these deficiencies, follow these strategies:

Regularly take a DHA & EPA vegan supplement

Soak and sprout your nuts and seeds before you eat them

Use vegan D3 to supplement your diet

Eat real food as much as possible and limit the intake of vegan junk

Take fermented soy or kale for vitamin K2

Eat sauerkraut, natto, and kimchi to aid digestion

Take iodine-rich foods such as seaweed to enhance selenium intake

For dry skin or feeling of unwell, take a zinc supplement

Eat foods rich in vitamin C to improve iron
absorption

Use one or all of these compounds:
creatine, carnosine, taurine

Add clams and oysters to your diet due to
their zinc and B-12 content

CHAPTER EIGHT

Mediterranean Keto Meal Plan

If you love Mediterranean foods, you can be part of the keto family too. Here is a sample to follow:

Monday

Breakfast: One or two slices of keto zucchini break with keto-friendly peanut butter, walnuts or homemade macadamia nut butter

Lunch: one serving maple shrimp salad

Dinner: one serving low-carb walnut crusted salmon

Extra dish: one or two servings of lemon roasted spicy broccoli

Tuesday

Breakfast: One or two servings of low-carb spiced baked eggs and cheesy hash

Lunch: One or two servings of lemony basil spread with salmon lettuce cups

Dinner: one serving of chicken tender lazone

Extra dish: a serving of raspberry pecan salad

Wednesday

Breakfast: One or two servings of vegan keto porridge

Lunch: Two servings of spinach watercress keto salad with chicken or fish for more protein

Dinner: one serving of zingy lemon fish

Extra dish: a serving of fiesta slaw and avocado lime salad

Thursday

Breakfast: use the leftover of the low-carb spiced baked eggs and cheesy hash, added to walnuts and one or two slices of keto zucchini bread

Lunch: two servings of egg salad stuffed avocado

Dinner: one or two servings of avocado-walnut pesto and zucchini ribbons with chicken or fish

Extra dish: one or two servings of roasted celery and macadamia cheese

Friday

Breakfast: eat the leftover of the low-carb spiced baked eggs and cheesy hash, added with one or two slices of keto zucchini bread with walnuts, and homemade macadamia nut or keto-friendly peanut butter

Lunch: one serving of maple shrimp salad

Dinner: one serving of low-carb walnut crusted salmon

Extra dish: raspberry pecan salad

Saturday

Breakfast: One or two servings of salmon benny breakfast bombs

Lunch: two servings of egg salad stuffed avocado

Dinner: one serving of zingy lemon fish

Extra dish: macadamia cheese and roasted celery

Sunday

Breakfast: One or two servings of vegan keto porridge

Lunch: One or two servings of salmon lettuce cups with lemony basil spread

Dinner: one or two servings of zucchini ribbons and avocado-walnut pesto

Extra dish: one or two servings of lemon roasted spicy broccoli

This is just a sample of what your Mediterranean keto meal plan should look like. It may not fulfill your personal needs but it is a good place to start. Always find a good keto calculator to customize your plan and reach your desired goals.

CHAPTER NINE

Things to Do Before Starting Keto

The meals recommended in a keto diet are simple but some people may find it hard to follow. The practice of moving from your normal intake of carbs to 50 grams per day may be a tough one. You can make the transition easier by following these steps.

Step 1: Plan Your Start Date

Remember it is not easy to go on a keto diet, so you will need good and proper planning. You need to understand what you are about to go into before you start. Choose the best day or week to start and try as much as possible to read up about the advantages and steps to the keto diet. Learn about the recommended foods and the ones you should avoid throughout the low-carb diet. Check your budget to see if you have what it takes it complete the journey. You will need enough resources to prepare the meals and recipes. Your family and friends need to know what you are up to, so you may need to inform them ahead. Tell them that your diet is about to change and you will no longer need pasta, rice, bread, and so on.

Step 2: Get Rid of Unwanted Carbs

If you will avoid the temptation of returning to your favorite foods, you will need to clear your cupboard and fridge of carbs. You should take them as far as possible to send them to a friend who is not yet on keto dieting. Do not assume that you can discipline yourself enough to resist the temptation of running back to them at the slightest difficulty of going through a low-carb diet. Once you make the mistake of falling into the trap of breaking keto rules, the harder the transition will be.

Step 3: Track Your Food with App

Keto diet is a diet that will demand a lot from you especially during the first week. You will be limiting the amount of carb intake to about 50 grams or less each day. For successful dieting, you will need to keep track of your food intake every day. Some of the good apps to use are My Plate, My Macros, and My Fitness Pal. With any of these trackers, you monitor and modify your meals to take the right amount of carbs, protein, and fat.

Step 4: Prepare for the First Two Weeks

The first two weeks will be the hardest you will experience in the keto journey. The reason is that your body needs time to adjust to the new dieting. It needs to use up all the previously stored carbs in the body before it can switch over to using ketones for fuel. You may or not experience some side effects or keto flu during this period. Some of the symptoms you will notice are insomnia, headaches, fatigue, cravings, and mood swings. Other keto flu you may notice are nausea, fruity-smelling breath, constipation, and increased urination.

There are signs that your body is responding positively to the transition from using carbs to using ketones for fuel. In this state, your body will soon start the fat burning process. The symptoms or side effects you experience will gradually disappear completely. Once these are gone and you do not cheat on the diet, you are not going to experience those symptoms ever again.

Step 5: Avoid Cheating on the Diet

You may have your way and cheat on other types of diet but not with a ketogenic diet. Keto is a form of diet that has a rule that you must follow through if you want to have maximum benefits. You cannot be on a keto and secretly take high-carb foods. If you do, you will quickly kick yourself out of the much-needed ketosis. And that will mean starting all over again and going through the keto flu you have dreaded once again. So do not think of cheating on this diet because it doesn't do you any good. If you feel like cheating, find something to take off the thought of it. You may go to the movies, visit a massage treatment center to make sure you don't fall for the high-carb bait.

Step 6: Make Keto a Lifestyle

When you plan your keto diet, make sure you are considering it long-term. Although you may not go on this diet forever, it is something that you would like to continue to keep your body healthy and strong. Some people plan it for a few weeks, worrying over the effects it is going to have on the body. They feel uncomfortable with the process of weight loss and then run back to their carbs even before they get started. What could be worse than losing weight and then regain weight again?

You will gain more and enjoy the diet more if you get comfortable with it and see it as a lifestyle in the long-term for as long as it lasts. This way, you eliminate the unnecessary worries and experience weight loss and other keto benefits.

Keep this in mind: you experience the benefits of this diet if you stay true to the dos and donts. Once you break them, you automatically wave goodbye to everything you have worked hard to achieve. You don't want to miss having reduced inflammation, a healthy heart, and lower blood pressure, do you?

Keto diet is good for those who are 50 years and above, and the benefits are more than just losing weight. Stick to the meal plan and don't think of breaking it in any way after a few weeks. Determine to make it a long-term practice until you see changes in all aspects of your health through this low-carb dieting.